HEALED:

Adjusting to Our New Normal

Dr. Jacqueline L. Jackson
&
Dr. Darryl S. Tukufu

Healed: Adjusting to Our New Normal
RiverHouse Publishing, LLC
1509 Madison Avenue
Memphis, TN 38104

All **RiverHouse, LLC** Titles, Imprints and Distributed Lines are available at special quantity discounts for bulk purchases for sales promotions, premiums, fund-raising and educational or institutional use.

First RiverHouse, LLC Paperback Publication: 7/31/2015

ISBN-10:
0996272542
ISBN-13:
978-0-9962725-4-4

www.riverhousepublishingllc.com

This book is dedicated to our Heavenly Father whose Word came to live in us more abundantly in our New Normal. We also dedicate this book to those who know God and who are suffering illness in their mind and/or body, realizing that spiritually, they are healed; and to those who do not know God but are open to hearing the Word of God as we share our testimony and offer them an open invitation to experience the Word as it is throughout our book. Finally, we dedicate our book to those that are yet to come.

Acknowledgments

I would like to say thanks to my mom Pearl, who sometimes worked on Sundays but showed me the way to Christ by making her children attend Sunday school and church, both in her company and during her absence. I also want to thank my husband, Ronald, for kindly encouraging me in many ways to continue writing, and for being supportive when I had to spend time away from home, monopolize the telephone, and spend endless hours on the computer, even though he knew I was "doing too much."

I want to thank Bishop Sherwood Carthen, former pastor of Bayside of South Sacramento, CA. He has gone on to glory, his sermons brought some truths to my life, and he took the time to listen to me when I needed it most. I give special thanks to my sister, Harriet, and my children, grandchildren and friends for their support and encouragement.

JLJ

Above all I want to thank my wife, Myra, and my youngest son, Khari. They supported me and encouraged me to pray and write, although it took me away from having date nights with Myra and watching action movies with Khari. I would also like to express my gratitude to the pastors and ministers of The House of the Lord (Akron, OH), Olivet Institutional Baptist Church (Cleveland, OH), Born Again Church (Nashville, TN), Greater Imani Church (Memphis, TN), and Mississippi Boulevard Christian Church (Memphis, TN) for their contributions to my spiritual upbringing and background.

DST

We would like to thank Pastor Gerald Lamont Thomas, Ph.D., of Shiloh Baptist Church, Plainfield, NJ, and Rev. James Mansel and his wife, Pamela, of Akron, OH, for their advice and guidance in writing this book. Additionally, we express our sincere gratitude to our editor, Donnetta Booker, and our publisher, RiverHouse Publishing.

JLJ & DST

Table of Contents

Introduction 1

Chapter One: Healing 5

Chapter Two: Jackie's Testimony 9

Chapter Three: Darryl's Testimony 13

Chapter Four: Sickness and Healing Scriptures 19

Chapter Five: Living Our New Normal 31

Works Cited 39

Appendix 41

About the Authors 43

Introduction

Let us begin with prayer. "Dear heavenly Father, we thank You for Your Word which we continue to hold on to as we experience our New Normal. It is Your Word God that continues to surround us with Your glory. We know it was, and continues to be, our faith in Your Word that our healing represents, for faith is the substance of things hoped for and the evidence of things not seen. We have come to know ourselves well as we live in our New Normal. Thank You for our healing. In Jesus' name we pray, Amen."

We met in Akron, OH in the early 1980's. We became good friends, but over the years our lives took different paths. We reconnected in 2013, and happened to mention various illnesses and diagnoses that we experienced. We decided to write a book from a Christian perspective to share how our illnesses have affected us and what that means for us as we now live our lives in a different state of awareness. Our purpose in writing this book is four-fold:

- To share with you our particular health challenges and diagnoses and their affect on us.
- To emphasize that after all is said and done, we are healed, and to explain what this healing means.
- To share Biblical references on sickness and healing that are encouraging to us. All scriptures referenced in this book are from the New International Version unless otherwise noted.

- To discuss our views on God's purpose for our illnesses, and how we can continue working for Christ via our New Normal.

We believe that Christ is surely the answer to all healing. In spite of the conditions of our body and mind in our New Normal, our soul, our spirit, is the most important ingredient in our healing. However, before we proceed, here are three points of context that will provide some perspective as you continue reading.

First and foremost, we stand on faith. 2 Corinthians 5:7 reminds us to "walk by faith, not by sight." Brent Barnett (2014 p. 1-2) expresses it well when he points out that,

"'Walk' speaks of how we live our lives, conduct ourselves, behave, and use the time and opportunities God has ordained for us. Walking 'by sight' speaks of choosing to live based upon how things naturally appear, feel, and seem at first glance. Those who walk by sight rely upon fleshly instincts and temporal pleasure to make decisions. They are concerned with the present rather than the eternal. Those who walk by faith are keenly aware of the temporal nature of this life and world, and their focus and hope is fixed upon heaven; walking by faith requires a willingness to suffer now, knowing that there will be no suffering later; walking by faith isn't only marked by suffering and sacrifice…it is also marked by service for the Lord; only by faith can we accomplish true spiritual victories through and in Christ."

Our walking in faith, or faith walk, leads us to believe that, in spite of our New Normal – which relates to the conditions of our body and mind – it is our soul, our spirit that stands out and is most important in our healing. Our faith allows us to accomplish true spiritual victories.

Second, let us characterize the term "New Normal." This term has been used in business and in psychology (Maisel, 2013). Most people perceive normal as being free from physical or mental disorders. However, the New Normal introduces something quite different. The Urban Dictionary (2013) provides an excellent definition by emphasizing that it is "the current state of being after some dramatic change has transpired," and that "the New Normal encourages one to deal with current situations rather than lamenting [about] what could have been." We are experiencing this "dramatic change," and we acknowledge our faith, hope, trust and belief in Jesus Christ, and that it is Him who assists us in dealing with our current life situations.

Third, this book is not designed as a scholarly piece. It is our testimony about how we are able to live in the face of illness as God shows us grace and mercy through His healing power, and how He continues to bless us as we live in our New Normal.

Chapter One:
Healing

Healing relates to our body, mind, and spirit. Oftentimes, when healing is considered two verses come to mind: Isaiah 53:5, "But he was pierced for our transgressions, he was crushed for our iniquities; the punishment that brought us peace was upon him, and by his wounds we are healed;" and 1 Peter 2:24, "He himself bore our sins in his body on the tree, so that we might die to sins and live for righteousness; by his wounds you have been healed." These verses indicate that Jesus, who was sinless, bore our sins and that He was the substitute, in His death, for our sins. The Hebrew word for healing is *rapha*, which means "to make thoroughly whole." The Greek word is *sozo* which means "save" and "heal." So His healing is our salvation. When Jesus died on the cross He saved us from our sins and made us whole in Him. We are spiritually healed through our salvation in Jesus Christ. His sacrificial gift of salvation brings well being to our mind, body, and spirit.

Our religion and faith teaches us that God can heal us in all ways, but He determines our healing outcome. Although we have received a spiritual healing based upon God's plans and promises for salvation and eternal life, we also believe that healing of our body and mind can occur if God so chooses. Our knowledge and faith go hand in hand as we recognize what we must actively do in trusting and believing God to receive His healing. Our knowledge of Him through our prayer lives, and our faith in His Will for our lives, began during our "healthy" times, and continues during our illnesses. Matthew 14:14 states, "When Jesus landed and saw a large crowd, he had compassion on them and healed their sick." We believe our spiritual healing is indicative of the same compassion and caring Jesus has for us that He had for the multitudes two thousand years ago. We recognize it was their faith in Christ that made them well, and it is our faith that makes and keeps us well daily as we adjust to living in our New Normal, which has been defined in the Introduction as "the current state of being after some dramatic change has transpired."

We believe that our illness and healing is an opportunity to

- Continue being faithful. Consider the woman with the issue of blood in Matthew 9:21, "She said to herself, 'If I only touch his cloak, I will be healed.'" She was healed because she acted in faith. By faith we trust and believe in God's favor for all our lives. It is our faith that makes us whole. Imagine what could happen if we showed this kind of faith in all aspects of our lives.

- Complete the purpose He has for our lives. We must continually seek Him daily through prayer and supplication to guide and instruct us on our journey rather than solely depending on ourselves and our personal beliefs.

- Offer hope to suffering people. Whenever and wherever possible, we share our testimonies of our healing and our New Normal with others who are living with illness, believing that it will help them as they go through their experiences.

- Strengthen our relationship with Him in love and obedience to His Word. We've been drawn closer to Him, and in our increased desire to please Him we have become more attuned to His voice when He speaks to us.

What a mighty God we serve!

It is important to understand and believe that we can still be healed even in this day and time. Practically every one of us knows someone who has been physically healed in some manner. We believe that we can be healed regardless of what others say. However, this healing will be a result of God's Will. James 4:14-15 states, "Why, you do not even know what will happen tomorrow. What is your life? You are a mist that appears for a little while and then vanishes. Instead, you ought to say, 'If it is the Lord's will, we will live and do this or that.'" He has to will it! His Will is what is paramount! All we have to do is make the decision to ask, trust, believe, and have faith in His Word that we are already healed.

Nevertheless, Jesus did not heal everyone He came in contact with. Healing was not the main point of His earthly ministry. He came to save the souls of sinners. The greater healing we receive is eternal life. Hebrews 9:15 states, "For this reason Christ is the mediator of a new covenant, that those who are called may receive the promised eternal inheritance..." This is why we say we are healed. For those of us who still have illnesses, we adjust to our New Normal and continue praising God.

Our illnesses have challenged us, shaped us, and drawn us even closer to God and to doing His will. The following verses say it best:

James 1:2-3
Consider it pure joy, my brothers and sisters, whenever you face trialsof many kinds, because you know that the testing of your faith produces perseverance.
2 Cor. 4:16
Therefore we do not lose heart. Though outwardly we are wasting away, yet inwardly we are being renewed day by day.

Thus, we acknowledge that we are spiritually healed and adjusting to our New Normal, which may be temporary, even in this world. However, if it is not God's Will to heal us in mind and body, we must accept His decision. We acknowledge Paul's plea to God when he wrote in 2 Corinthians 12 about the "thorn in his flesh." In verses 8 and 9 he stated, "Three times I pleaded with the Lord to take it away. But he said to me, 'My grace is sufficient for you, for my power is made perfect in weakness.'" In verse 10, which is very instructive for us, Paul says, "...for Christ's sake, I delight in weaknesses, in insults, in hardships, in persecutions, in difficulties. For when I am weak, then I am strong." We believe Paul is telling us to exercise our belief in our healing rather than give power to our ailments and any associated challenges. We accept the blessings God has bestowed upon us, and praise God joyfully for loving us in His way and allowing us to live healed and adjusting to a New Normal. All of this is to the glory of God!

Chapter Two:
Jackie's Testimony

~*My Christian Walk*~

I am most proud of growing up in the church and maintaining a close relationship with God. This is not to say that I did not go astray. My husband often tells me, "I am so glad God saved your soul." I began my walk with Christ at an early age, attending St. John C.M.E. Church in Akron, OH, where I sang in the Rosebud Choir in a pink, angelic-looking robe. I mouthed the words of the songs because I couldn't carry a tune in my hip pocket. When I was older, I joined Providence Baptist Church and continued my membership at various Baptist churches over the years. I joined Ingleside Presbyterian Church while living in San Francisco, where I was active with the youth, became President of the Women's Auxiliary, and was ordained as an Elder. My family and I moved to Sacramento and joined Bayside of South Sacramento (BOSS), where I am a member of the Local Organizing Committee and a past member of the Ghana Water Project.

~*My Health Challenges*~

As far as I know, two women in my family suffered strokes. My mother passed away from a massive stroke on December 15, 1995. My older sister suffered two strokes in 2005, which left her debilitated on her right side, and a minor stroke in 2013 leaving no consequences. On December 19, 2012, I lost consciousness for a few seconds, or so I think, while I was typing on the computer. When I regained consciousness, I went upstairs to use the restroom. As I walked toward the bedroom, I became unable to move my body on my right side. My husband drove me to the emergency room, and to my amazement the doctor ordered me to stay overnight.

The next day I was told I had suffered a Transient Ischemic Attack (TIA), or a mini stroke, where blood flow is interrupted when an artery supplying the brain with blood becomes blocked, causing a brain infarction (National Institute of Neurological Disorders and Stroke, 1996). I was astonished by this diagnosis because I had not previously suffered from headaches or any serious illnesses that would lead me to believe that I was at risk for a stroke. In fact, I felt good most of the time. I asked the doctor what were the causes of TIA, and he said that basically being an African-American is a factor. A TIA begins similarly to a stroke with symptoms that develop over a few minutes. They may include loss of strength sensation on one side of the body, problems with speech and language, or changes in vision or balance (Stroke at a Glance, American Stroke Association, 1999). The TIA clears up and leaves no noticeable symptoms or deficits. It is, however, a warning sign that there is risk for a more serious and debilitating stroke. Women have fewer strokes than men, but more women than men die from having suffered a stroke because women are usually older when they have them. To add insult to injury, I was also diagnosed with Hypercholesterolemia, or high cholesterol. My love of fried chicken, potato chips and potato salad had caught up with me.

After returning home, I began reading <u>Stroke at a Glance</u>, the booklet I was given while in the hospital. I did additional research on strokes at the library, and I browsed various websites such as The American Heart Association. One of the things I learned is that ischemic strokes usually occur first thing in the morning. I found that to be particularly interesting, as my first stroke had occurred around 9:30 am.

On January 11, 2013, I awakened with blindness in my right eye. I got an appointment that morning with an ophthalmologist. She referred me to a neuro-ophthalmologist, a doctor who specializes in diagnosing optic nerve related issues. On January 22, 2013, I received a diagnosis of Primary Optic Disc Edema (PODE), which caused permanent partial blindness. More simply put – I had a stroke in my right eye.

On January 28, 2013, I visited the neuro-ophthalmologist again because I was suffering from increased tearing, yellow floaters and dull eye pressure in my left eye – very similar to what I had experienced with my right eye. I was diagnosed with Non-Arteritic Anterior Ischemic Optic Neuropathy, or NAION – a stroke in my left eye. I was told there is a possibility I could also lose sight in my left eye. I then underwent several tests which included a visual field exam, a brain MRI, computerized Ophthalmic imaging of the optic nerve and the retina, and Fundus photography. None of these procedures were able to determine when the strokes in either eye actually occurred.

My next visit was to my neurologist. He took an Electroencephalogram (EEG), where electrodes were attached to my head to check for seizures. He stated that this should have been done during my stay in the hospital. During our visit, he was able to define some of my earlier symptoms, which occurred two months prior to my first stroke, as seizures. He discussed seizure medication, and informed me that I would need to take it if I wanted to drive. I have friends and relatives who take medicine for seizures, and I am quite familiar with the side effects. I asked the neurologist if he would advise his daughter or wife to take this medicine if they had the same medical summation as me. He told me no. I responded, "And neither will I."

Chapter Three:
Darryl's Testimony

~My Christian Walk~

I attended church sporadically during my younger years, but did so mainly using it as a social outlet. If girls were there, that was the place I wanted to be. From eighteen years of age and for the next thirteen years, I was agnostic and atheistic. I did not believe in Christianity mainly because I felt that it was not logical, with respect to a virgin birth, and that it was Eurocentric because all the biblical images I saw were white. The closest I came to a spiritual focus was following Kawaida, a philosophy developed by Dr. Maulana Karenga, the founder of Us Organization and Kwanzaa. Kawaida, in part, was based on African customs being reasonably applied to the experience of black people in America. However, at thirty-one years of age, I was baptized by Bishop Joey Johnson, pastor of The House of The Lord, in Akron, OH. I approached Christianity from a different point of view. Being an analytical and logical individual, I had to comprehend Christianity by first obtaining an intellectual understanding. Bishop Johnson gave me a copy of Josh McDowell's book, <u>Evidence That Demands A Verdict</u>, and it had such an impact on me that I finally came to believe in our faith. This book used secular evidence, historical sources, and specific documented archaeological discoveries to demonstrate the trustworthiness of scripture. One thing that particularly stuck with me was the assertion, "If Jesus was not

God, then He deserved an Oscar (McDowell 1979, p. 79)."

On Sunday, June 2, 2002, I experienced the Holy Spirit during the worship service at Born Again Church in Nashville, TN. While the choir was singing, I began speaking in tongues. On that following Thursday, June 6th, while shaving my head, I stopped in my tracks when I looked in the mirror and saw a large swatch of blood on the top of my head. I thought I had a large cut so I looked down, wrung out my facecloth and looked up again to wipe the blood away. However, there was no blood! I grabbed a hand mirror and looked all over my head and, let me emphasize again, *there was no blood!* I freaked out! I saw one of our pastors later that day and told him what happened. He stated, "God was covering you!" That did it for me. I promised God that I was going to get further into His Word. The next time a minister in training class started, I, joined by my wife, was there.

~My Health Challenges~

I used to think that illnesses were what others had. I believed that no major illness was going to occur in my life because I worked out about five days a week and I am a quasi-vegetarian – eliminating pork and beef from my diet and sticking with fish and poultry. Also, at this writing, my mother is twenty-two years older than me, and my father, who passed away in November 2013, was twenty-three years older than me. Given that both have dealt with their own illnesses and made it well into their eighties, with my mother still going strong, I figured I would have some longevity.

Nonetheless, in the last five years I have been diagnosed with a medium hiatal hernia, plantar fasciitis (PF) accompanied by superficial thrombosis, and Parkinson's Disease (PD). The hernia occurred around 2009, but it took a year for the diagnosis. I visited quite a few doctors; a general practitioner, an allergist, an ear, nose and throat specialist, and then a gastroenterologist. The picture of my chest cavity illustrated that I have the most common type of hernia – the sliding-hiatal hernia where the stomach and the section of the esophagus that joins the stomach slide up into the chest through the hiatus. However, what was so annoying was that my symptoms were linked to Gastro Esophageal Reflux Disease (GERD). There are certain foods I used to eat, such as tomatoes, apples, oranges, pineapples, and heavy milk products, that I can no longer digest as they produce acid reflux.

I also had a terrible, dry cough for a year. No matter what I took, the cough continued morning, noon, and night. Nothing that was prescribed worked. After numerous coughing spells, and loss of weight, I sometimes felt that death would have been better than what I was experiencing. Yes, I know, many of us men just can't stand much pain. Then one day while in Walgreens, I was led (it had to be God) to purchase their brand of acid reducer. The ingredients were similar to what had been previously prescribed for me, but it was labeled "maximum strength" so I purchased it anyway. My cough went away almost immediately. Just think, a whole year of consistent coughing was finally over. That simple medicine is still helping me today.

In 2009, I experienced PF in my right foot. The plantar fascia is the connective tissue on the bottom surface of our feet which causes a great deal of pain when inflamed. I had to wear a boot cast and a night splint, and was on crutches for nearly three weeks. In 2011, I experienced it again, but this time it was my left foot. Within a month of alleviating this pain, I experienced a great deal of swelling in my left foot. I went to a podiatrist and he referred me right away to a glandular surgeon. I was diagnosed with superficial thrombophlebitis – inflammation of a vein caused by a blood clot in the vein that runs from the inside of my left foot nearly up to my knee. Today, the swelling comes and goes, particularly when my body heats up, and also because I have varicose veins, which are prone to inflammation.

Sometime during 2011, I began experiencing unusual things with my body, but charged it to becoming older, and possibly a result of PF. My body movement was not quite the same. I felt extra stiff and had some problems with limbering up and doing my exercises. I even had a few colleagues remark that I either "walked like a zombie" or "walked like a soldier with no swing to my arms." I dismissed this as having good posture because back in the day, my mother had me walk around the house with a book on my head. Then at the end of the summer in 2012, I remarked to my general practitioner that I had been experiencing shaking – an involuntary tremor in my left hand that was difficult to stop. He suggested that I see a neurologist.

On September 18, 2012, I was checked by a neurologist and diagnosed with Parkinson's Disease (PD). All I knew about PD was that Michael J. Fox and Muhammad Ali had it. The following day I had a brain MRI and started on some medication. The doctor told me if the MRI results were all right and the medicine helped my symptoms, this would verify the diagnosis. After two weeks I had a follow-up appointment where the diagnosis was confirmed as my symptoms had improved and the MRI results had come back negative.

I then began to read all I could about this disease. I learned that it is a degenerative disorder of the central nervous system with an early stage, when life could be fairly normal; a moderate stage when you need to accept help; and a late stage when you reach the point of a serious disability (Tagliati 2007, p. 38-40). Symptoms related to PD, which I have experienced, include rigid posture, slowed or slurred speech, incontinence, anxiety, small and/or cramped handwriting, a tremor present in one limb, and sleep disturbances. My current symptoms, as of spring 2014, are in the early stage, with a few in the moderate stage. From talks with my doctor and through my own research, I know that if my disease progresses, I would need to prepare to rely more on others for some assistance. I continue to believe, with respect to my healing – mind, body, and soul – that prayer will help me to overcome, and bring about healing in mind and body; as I am already healed with respect to my soul, my spirit.

Chapter Four:
Sickness and Healing Scriptures

JACKIE

Sickness is discussed throughout the Bible. As I read the various situations where the persons described are healed of their sicknesses, the word "service" comes to mind. The very act of healing is a service in itself. In Matthew 15:30-39, Jesus not only healed the multitudes, He continued to serve them by feeding them as well. Conversely, there are instances where healing inspires the spirit of service in others. For example, Mark 2:1-5 tells how four men lowered a paralyzed man through the roof of a home where Jesus was appearing to receive healing from Jesus. Their desire to help their friend to be healed was so strong that they went to extraordinary measures to get him to Jesus. In Luke 8:2, Jesus healed a demon possessed woman named Mary Magdalene. She then served Jesus as she followed Him "and cared for his needs" (Mark 15:40-41), and comforted Him at His crucifixion (John 19:25).

Being well in body, mind and spirit incorporates our ability to love and serve God with all our heart, our soul, our strength, and our mind, and to love others as we love ourselves (Luke 10:27). Loving, and serving, others may not be an easy task, but it gets easier as we trust God to keep His promises to us. This promise helps me when it comes to my body and soul. God says in Isaiah 57:19, "'...Peace, peace to those far and near,' says the Lord. 'And I will heal them.'" What a way to ease all that anxiety and anxiousness, because no matter where I go, near or far, I am at peace with my suffering and I am healed from my sicknesses.

God healed us so that we might continue to be good soldiers in His army. The battlefield on which we serve is new every day of our lives. When you arise in the morning, before you think about the difficulties that lay ahead, or that husband or wife who upset you last night, think of the promise of joy God gives us in Psalm 30:5, "For his anger lasts only a moment, but his favor lasts a lifetime; weeping may remain for a night, but rejoicing comes in the morning."

Recently I watched President Barack Obama present the Medal of Honor to a soldier who was wounded in battle, yet continued to serve his fellow soldiers. He ran back and forth through gunfire to take them ammunition as they were under a tremendous attack from the enemy. If that wasn't enough, he ran through a barrage of bullets to help his fellow soldiers carry their wounded comrade to the medical post before receiving attention for his own wounds. His story reminded me that there is always a service for us to give no matter when, no matter how, no matter what. God will give us support to handle anything. We are never alone. In 1 Corinthians 10:13, He promises us that even in the midst of temptation, He "will also make the way of escape, that you may be able to endure it." Thanks to Bishop Carthen, my former pastor at Bayside of South Sacramento, I have come to understand that this scripture has nothing to do with what was told to me in the past, "He will not put more on you than you can bear." It means as it says, "And God is faithful; he will not let you be *tempted* beyond what you can bear." I was tempted to hold onto things that made me sick.

I made myself sick by taking things personally, refusing to forgive others when they hurt me, and failing to forgive myself of my own sinful past. Instead, I would ponder for long periods of time, battling to let go of stuff and remain sick. I thank God that I embraced His message in 1 Corinthians 10:13, realizing that He wants me well. I also read a book entitled, <u>The Four Agreements</u> by Don Miguel Ruiz. His statement, "by taking things personally you set yourself up to suffer for nothing (p 62)," helped me realize that I needed to trust in God and not in people or myself. In Him I can do anything.

Hold in your heart the following scriptures on sickness:

FAVOR/WRATH/HUMILITY

The following passage demonstrates to me how I must humble myself before God with a clean heart. This scripture encourages me to relinquish having a proud heart, and continue to be faithful with my walk with Christ.

2 Chron 32:24-26
In those days Hezekiah became ill and was at the point of death.

He prayed to the Lord, who answered him and gave him a miraculous sign. But Hezekiah's heart was proud and he did not respond to the kindness shown him; therefore the Lord's wrath was on him and on Judah and Jerusalem. Then Hezekiah repented of pride of his heart, as did the people of Jerusalem; therefore the Lord's wrath did not come upon them during the days of Hezekiah.

OBEDIENCE

The following passages demonstrate to me that obediently listening to God assures me and my children life. Now, I spend more time listening to God so that I can hear His voice over mine.

Deut. 30:19- 20

This day I call heaven and earth as witnesses against you that I have set before life and death, blessings and curses. Now choose life, so that you and your children may live and that you may love the Lord your God, listen to his voice, and to hold to him. For the Lord is your life, and he will give you many years in the land he swore to give to your fathers, Abraham, Isaac and Jacob.

1 John 3:22

…and receive from him anything we ask, because we obey his commands and do what pleases him.

RESTORATION

In 2 Kings 4:18-37, a story is told of a Shunammite woman whose young son cried out to his father that he had a terrible headache. The child died. However, his mother's faith was strong. She appealed to her friend, the Prophet Elisha, and he was able to return her son to life. Like the story of the Shunammite woman, the following passages remind me how God is able to give back what has been taken away.

Psalm 41:1-3

Blessed is he who has regard for the weak; the Lord delivers him in times of trouble. The Lord will protect him and preserve his life; he will bless him in the land and not surrender him to the desire of his foes. The Lord will sustain him on his sickbed and restore him from his bed of illness.

Luke 4:18

The spirit of the Lord is on me because he has anointed me to preach good news to the poor. He has sent me to proclaim freedom for the prisoners and the recovery of sight for the blind, to release the oppressed.

FEAR THE LORD FOR HE IS MERCIFUL!

I chose the following passages because God has shown mercy upon me for my healing. I realize that everything we need from God is only a prayer away.

Psalm 6:2

Be merciful to me, Lord, for I am faint; O Lord, heal me, for my bones are in agony.

Mark 5:9-15

..."My name is Legion," he replied, "for we are many."...The demons begged Jesus, "Send us among the pigs; allow us to run into them." He gave them permission, and the evil spirits came out [of the man] and went into the pigs. The herd rushed down the steep bank into the lake and were drowned. Those tending the pigs ran off and reported this in the town and the countryside, and the people went out to see what had happened. When they came to Jesus, they saw the man who had been possessed by the legion of demons, sitting there dressed and in his right mind; and they were afraid.

Luke 4:40
When the sun was setting, the people brought to Jesus all who had various kinds of sicknesses, and laying his hands on each one, he healed them.

Luke 10: 8-9 "When you enter a town and are welcomed, eat what is set before you. Heal the sick who are there and tell them, 'The Kingdom of God is near you."

A TIME FOR PRAISE

The following passage demonstrates how God sometimes gives us more than we can imagine for ourselves. This man asked only for alms as he sat at the temple gate called Beautiful, yet he received healing in his body.

Acts 3:6-8
Then Peter said, "Silver or gold I do not have, but what I do have I give you. In the name of Jesus Christ of Nazareth, walk." Taking him by the right hand, he helped him up, and instantly the man's feet and ankles became strong. He jumped to his feet and began to walk. Then he went with them into the temple courts, walking and jumping, and praising God.

HEALED

The following scriptures speak personally to me the reasons why I know I am healed and live a more healthy and vigorous life after having endured my strokes. I am healed within my whole self.

Psalm 30:2
Oh Lord my God, I called to you for help and you healed me.

Psalm 107:20
He sent forth his word and healed them; he rescued them from the grave.

Jeremiah 17:14
Heal me, O Lord, and I shall be healed;...for you are my praise.

Luke 13:11-12
And a woman was there who had been crippled by a spirit for eighteen years. She was bent over and could not straighten up at all. When Jesus saw her, he called her forward and said to her, "Woman, you are set free from your infirmity."

James 5:16
Therefore, confess your sins to each another, and pray for each other, so that you may be healed.

3 John 1:2
Dear friend, I pray that you may enjoy good health and that all may go well with you, even as your soul is getting along well.

DARRYL
In both the Old and New Testaments, a number of individuals had varying ailments. Although I'm currently dealing with my own set of ailments, my faith is not diminished. There are sixteen verses that I find comfort-

ing, and are particularly helpful as I adjust to my New Normal. These first three verses reinforce my faith and belief that I can be delivered from whatever ails me.

Exodus 23:25
Worship the Lord your God, and his blessing will be on your food and water. I will take away sickness from among you.

Matthew 6:33
But seek first his kingdom and his righteousness, and all these things will be given to you as well.

Psalm 34:19
A righteous man may have many troubles, but the Lord delivers him from them all.

I find that "praise" scripture helps move me through the day. My favorite is:

Psalm 103:2-3
Praise the Lord, my soul, and forget not all his benefits—who forgives all your sins and heals all your diseases.

There are times when I find that I am my best cheerleader, being moved to rejoice and applaud my progress by this encouraging and wise scripture:

Proverbs 17:22
A cheerful heart is good medicine, but a crushed spirit dries up the bones.

I find this following quote in Isaiah particularly helpful because at times I have suffered from anxiety and
depression because of illness. This is the case for many
people who are dealing with illness, and some may have
even felt that they would rather go and be with Jesus
than go through what they are experiencing. If it's His
Will to call them home now, it will happen. But if it's
His Will for them to adjust to their New Normal, this
verse can provide hope:

Isaiah 41:10
So do not fear, for I am with you; do not be dis-
mayed, for I am your God. I will strengthen you and
help you; I will uphold you with my righteous right hand.

Regardless of the diagnoses by my various doctors,
it's not over until the Lord says it is. Therefore, I get
excited when I quote the following two verses:

Jeremiah 29:11
For I know the plans I have for you, declares the
Lord, plans to prosper you and not to harm you, plans to
give you hope and a future.

Jeremiah 30:17
But I will restore you to health and heal your
wounds, declares the Lord,

I have participated in various workshops on personal
growth and development, and health and healing where
one or more individuals would blurt out, "Why me?" or,
"Why me Lord?" When asked whether or not they
prayed or asked for healing, they answered, "Maybe a

couple of times." Their response indicates to me that they most likely didn't believe they would be healed even when they were praying for it. If we can't believe the following scripture in Matthew, then we are folks with little faith:

Matthew 7:7-8
Ask and it will be given to you; seek and you will find; knock and the door will be opened to you. For everyone who asks receives; he who seeks finds; and to him who knocks, the door will be opened.

There is also hope in the following four verses. Although we know that Jesus did not heal everyone, He did heal all those who were brought to Him, or requested it of Him.

Matthew 9:35
Jesus went through all the towns and villages, teaching in their synagogues, preaching the good news of the kingdom and healing every disease and sickness.

Matthew 14:14
When Jesus landed and saw a large crowd, he had compassion on them and healed their sick.

Acts 5:16
Crowds gathered also from the towns around Jerusalem, bringing their sick and those tormented by evil spirits, and all of them were healed.

Acts 10:37-38
You know what has happened throughout Judea, beginning in Galilee after the baptism that John preached—how God anointed Jesus of Nazareth with the Holy Spirit and power and how he went around doing good and healing all who were under the power of the devil, because God was with him.

Throughout this book we have emphasized the importance of faith. Faith is also evident when a follower of Christ maintains an illness or disease; equivalent to what we say is "adjusting to our New Normal." It is probably stated best in scripture when Paul complained to the Lord three times about "the thorn in his flesh" which could not be relieved through prayer. Paul concluded that the Lord didn't move on his request because it was a way to keep him from becoming conceited.

2 Cor. 12:9-10
But he said to me, my grace is sufficient for you, for my power is made perfect in weakness.Therefore, I will boast all the more gladly about my weaknesses, so that Christ's power may rest on me.

The following verses speak to those who are ordained, in this case the elders, to assist and serve the afflicted:

James 5:14-15
Is any one of you sick? He should call the elders of the church to pray over him and anoint him with oil in the name of the Lord. And the prayer offered in faith

will make the sick person well; the Lord will take him up if he has sinned, he will be forgiven.

My final scripture is similar to a few others, but the word "confidence" stands out to me. I see confidence as synonymous with faith.

1 John 5:14
This is the confidence we have in approaching God: that if we ask anything according to his will, he hears us.

Chapter Five:
Living Our New Normal

We stated in the Introduction that there were four things we would do. First, share our diagnoses to show that you can be a healthy individual at one time in your life, but if it's God's Will, things can, and will, change.

Second, we emphasized that in spite of our present state, we are still healed. We believe in God's supernatural, spiritual healing – eternal life. We also believe in physical healing, as we know and have heard of individuals who were diagnosed with cancer and later determined cancer-free. We see it with those who have experienced serious leg injuries and were told they would not walk again, in spite of therapy; yet after a period of time find they have no problem with walking or running. However, God's spiritual healing is the greatest healing we can receive because:

- We rely on God to make us well, a wellness that permeates the aspects of our total being – mind, body, and spirit.

- God is perfect in our weaknesses. As He says in 2 Corinthians 12:9, "My grace is sufficient for you, for my power is made perfect in weakness,"

- We have the whole armor of God to protect us. Ephesians 6:13-17 emphasizes this full armor which includes the belt of truth, the breastplate of righteousness, gospel shoes, the shield of faith, the helmet of salvation, and the sword of the Spirit.

- We give life to the spiritual energy transferred to us by the crucifixion of Jesus Christ, "...by His wounds you have been healed." (1 Peter 2:24)

In the New Normal we live to do God's work because we recognize and appreciate more than ever His gift of eternal life. When illness comes, our surrendering to His Will is when we are healed. We accept His blessing of healing. The Father just gives it to us because He loves us, His children, so much. He gave His only begotten Son so that we "may have life, and have it to the full." (John 10:10)

Third, we provided scriptural references that have helped us adjust to our New Normal. We can definitely attest to the power of the Word and its impact on us.

Fourth, we will now expound upon why we believe we are experiencing our current health challenges. We believe that our present suffering shapes us into the type of people that God wants working for Him. James 1:2-4 tells us to "Consider it pure joy, my brothers, whenever you face trials of many kinds, because you know that the testing of your faith produces perseverance. Perseverance must finish its work so that you may be mature and complete, not lacking anything."

Additionally, Herb Vander Lugt (1997 p. 30-31) states, "Yes, God wants you well. God's Word provides assurances and promotes a way of life that is conducive to physical and psychological wellness. It does so in at least nine ways: 1. it brings relief from the heavy burden of guilt (Psalm 32:1-3; Romans 5:1). 2. It provides the power to release inner bitterness caused by an unforgiving spirit (Matthew 6:12, 14-15; Ephesians 4:32). 3. It promotes a positive view toward our body, assuring us that the Holy Spirit lives in it (1 Corinthians 6:19), in that it is destined for resurrection (1 Corinthians 15). 4. It teaches that sexual expression is both safe and satisfying within the bonds of marriage (1 Corinthians 7:1-5; Hebrews 13:4). 5. It provides grace for single believers, enabling them to live a happy and fulfilled life (1 Corinthians 7:7-8, 32, 39-40). 6. It is marked by hope- a buoyant confidence about the future (Romans 8:31-39). 7. It assures us that we are members of a select community-the body of Christ in which each person fills a special roll for the mutual benefit of all (Romans 12:3-8; 1 Corinthians 12:1-31). 8. It fosters a unique relationship with God so that we can come to Him as our Father in an attitude of expectancy and ask Him for healing when we are sick (Matthew 7:7-11; Romans 8:15; James 5:14-15). 9. It enables us to rejoice even when we suffer pain (Acts 5:14; 2 Corinthians 4:16-18). God wants you well. He allows illness and pain only when He can use them for your good. And He is going to see to it that you will be well for all eternity. Believing this will promote your good health."

Yes, there may be times when we resort back to, "Why me, Lord, why me?" However, we must choose to stand by the following: "Therefore, we do not lose heart. Though outwardly we are wasting away, yet inwardly we are being renewed day by day. For our light and momentary troubles are achieving for us an eternal glory that far outweighs them all. So we fix our eyes not on what is seen, but on what is unseen. For what is seen is temporary, but what is unseen is eternal." (2 Corinthians 4:16-18)

JACKIE

In my New Normal, I have learned to become less anxious; whereas before I would get frustrated and irritated with things and people. I called it "getting on my nerves," and reacted in a very ugly manner. I now pray more, and quietly hum the songs I heard my mom sing. *Pass me not o gentle Savior...* It causes me to rest, and it helps me to listen to my body when it tells me to let things go.

I also find myself becoming more patient and more easily forgiving of others. I would often dwell on things people did or said that were contrary to my beliefs. But who am I to judge? I now spend much more time in God's Word, along with others who wish to join with me.

I've made some specific life changes in the New Normal that are directly related to the loss of sight in my right eye. When I awaken each morning, I have to adjust to my partial vision. Therefore, I wait for my eye to allow me to see. Some days I have less vision than others. When reaching for an object in a dark place, I must look for it twice because the first time I look, it is not there. I have learned to use my right arm to judge distance between myself, people, and objects, and to balance myself when I use the stairs. When walking outside with others, for my safety and comfort, I ask them to walk on my right side. Sometimes my husband walks on my right side when we are in crowded areas and near buildings.

My New Normal has required me to make additional lifestyle changes and adjustments as follows:

- My speech is slurred. Therefore, now when I speak to people, I speak more slowly.

- Sometimes when I think I am humming a song or speaking softly, others tell me I am speaking or singing loudly. I apologize and begin to pay more attention to my singing or speaking.

- I have always taken much pride in my hand-writing. Now I do a lot of printing because I tend to lose letters. For instance, while writing the word "example," it becomes "axample," and "anxiousness" becomes "aous."

- I have memory lapses and have to write down nearly everything that is important for me to remember. Many people tell me it comes with age.

- Because I cannot drive, I am humbled to ask people to take me places. My husband calls it "driving Miss Daisy." I call it an occasion to go places when others are ready.

- Sometimes by body attempts to surge into action like a Hemi engine. In the past, I drove my body like that. Now, I have to talk my body into driving like a fashionable Model T Ford. It takes a moment for my body to adjust, but it's worth the wait.

- I continue to research my TIA, my PODE, and my NAION, and I attend stroke support group meetings twice a month.

- I have exchanged hatefulness for hopeful-ness.

DARRYL

I am approaching two years since I was diagnosed with PD, and I thank God that I am still here and doing well. I read my Bible daily, particularly focusing on the "Daily Bread." I am eating properly (although I still have problems staying away from deserts), I take my medication daily, along with a blend that includes acai berry and whey protein, and I exercise on a regular basis. I lift light weights about three times a week, and on alternating days I do Tai Chi or line dancing. I am also on the treadmill at least five days a week. I have very little body fat and try to maintain my weight between 180-185 pounds. Additionally, my work is not affected by this disease.

Nonetheless, there continues to be a New Normal that has caused me to make some adjustments:

- I find myself becoming more calm and patient, which is extremely difficult for one who's known for being in a hurry most of the time.
- Sometimes it takes me a while to get in and out of cars because I feel out of balance. I take my time, move more slowly, and make sure that I am steady before proceeding.
- Something simple like buttoning my shirts and putting on a jacket or coat is difficult. It requires more effort than it used to. There are times that I have had to ask my wife for assistance. The next step will be to attach velcro to the top button area of my dress shirts and cuffs.

- I have a pretty regular tremor in my left hand. For relief I sometimes use a small squeeze ball, put my hand in my pocket, or, if sitting, place my hand on my thigh. Sometimes I hold my left hand with my right hand. If someone should ask what I'm doing, I already have a response, "Pardon me, but Parkinson's Disease is trying to control me and I won't let it."

- Occasionally my body will shift back and forth between regular movement and stiffness. I try to focus on this long enough to speed up my gait or add some additional movement to my body.

- Jackie indicated that she sometimes speaks more loudly than she believes she is. Just the opposite occurs with me. I think I am speaking loudly and people will tell me that they can hardly hear me. I try to be more conscious of this and speak, as I believe, more audibly.

- I find myself getting even more into the Word as I feel challenged to do so. Memorization does not seem to be as easy today as it was years ago, but I am committed to staying on this path.

JACKIE AND DARRYL

Our New Normal has changed us day by day. We have a stronger dependence upon God, and a closer relationship with Him. We realize now more than ever that we must be servants to His Word and to His people. Our New Normal has also given us valuable blessings in areas of personal growth that we otherwise would not have received.

Our hearts are filled with the joy of being one of many people who have been chosen to receive His healing power. We certainly recognize the probability of more health issues in the future; however, we stand upon our healing experiences, our knowledge of Him, and the power of His Word. He healed us once. He can do it over and over again. God wants us well!

As we close let us pray: "Dear God, we thank You for giving us Your Spirit that led us to write this book and give personal testimonies on being healed and living in our New Normal. We thank you for our families and friends that continue to show us love and concern via their prayers, their telephone calls, emails, and visits. We thank You for the doctors you placed in our lives and pray that they continue to make the right decisions that will help keep us growing in faith as we pray for total healing. We pray that the readers of this book will witness Your blessings upon our lives because we stepped out on faith to claim our healing and live fully, rather than waste away living a life less than the one promised to us through Your Son's crucifixion. In Your Son Jesus' name we pray, Amen, and Amen."

Works Cited

American Stroke Association, a Division of American Heart Association (1999). "Stroke at a Glance." Dallas, Texas: American Stroke Association.

Barnett, Brent (2014). "The Real Meaning of Walking By Faith." Retrieved on February 27, 2014 from www.relevantbibleteaching.com

Lugt, Herb Vander (1997:30-31). *Does God Want Me Well?* Grand Rapids, Michigan: R.B.C.Ministries.

Maisal, Eric (2013, February). Rethinking Psychology: The New Normal. *Psychology Today*.Retrieved on February 15, 2014 from http://www.psychology.com/blog/rethinking-__psychology/201302/the-new-normal

McDowell, Josh, *Evidence That Demands A Verdict: Historical Evidences for the Christian Faith* (1979), San Bernardino, CA: Here's Life Publishers, Inc

National Institute of Neurological Disorders and Stroke (1996). *Stroke.* Bethesda,Maryland: National Institute of Health, NIAH Pub. No. 99-2222

Ruiz, Don Miguel (1997:53-66). *The Four Agreements: A Practical Guide to PersonalFreedom (A Toltec Wisdom Book).* San Rafael, California: Amber-Allen Publishing, Inc.

Tagliati, Michele, MD, Guten, Gary N., MD, Horne, MA (2007). *Parkinson's DiseaseFor Dummies*. Hoboken, N.J.:Wiley Publishing Company.

Urban Dictionary (2013, March 1). Urban Dictionary. New Normal. Retrieved on February 15,2014 from http://www.urbandictionary.com/define/php?term=New%20normal

Appendix

Scriptural References Used by Jackson and Tukufu

Old Testament

Exodus 23:25
Deuteronomy 30:19-20
2 Kings 4:18-37
2 Chronicles 32:24-26
Psalm 6:2
Psalm 30:2
Psalm 30:5
Psalm 34:19
Psalm 41:1-3

Psalm 103:2-3
Psalm 107:20
Proverbs 17:22
Isaiah 41:10
Isaiah 53:5
Isaiah 57:19
Jeremiah 17:14
Jeremiah 29:11
Jeremiah 30:17

New Testament

Matthew 6:33
Matthew 7:7-8
Matthew 9: 21, 35
Matthew 14:14
Matthew 15:30-39
Mark 2:1-5
Mark 5:9-15
Mark 15:40-41
Luke 4:18, 40
Luke 8:2
Luke 10:8-9, 27
Luke 13:11-12
John 10:10
John 19:25
Acts 3:6-8

Acts 5:16
Acts 10:37-38
1 Corinthians 10:13
2 Corinthians 4:16-18
2 Corinthians 5:7
2 Corinthians 12:8-10
Ephesians 6:13-17
Hebrews 9:15
James 1:2-4
James 4:14-15
James 5:14-16
1 Peter 2:24
1 John 3:22
1 John 5:14
3 John 1:2

About the Authors

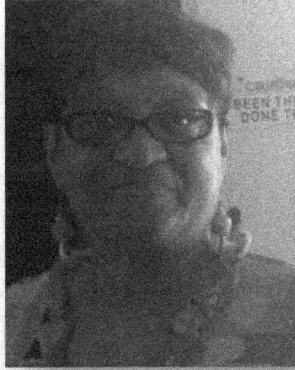

Dr. Jacqueline L. Jackson

Jackie held membership and offices in several Black cultural organizations. She was a member of the Society for Cooperative Improvement of African Americans (SCIA), the National Black Political Assembly (NBPA), the National Black Independent Political Party (NBIPP), the National Black Women's Leadership Conference (NBWLC), Akron, OH Chapter, and the Afrikan National Rites of Passage Kollective (ANROPUK).

She continued her community involvement by working with children and families as a social worker at Stark Social Workers' Network and Chou Weusi Saturday School.

She co-founded the P.I.E.C.E. Tutorial Program and Sisters With a Vision (SWV), and she was the Tutorial Supervisor at the Police Community Dialogue.

She was an employment specialist at the Private Industry Council (PIC) and also co-facilitated workshops at two Ohio Baptist Convention Women's Conferences.

Jackie completed her doctoral program at The University of Akron and held positions at this institution and Niagara University in Niagara Falls, New York. She moved to San Francisco, California to remarry her husband, Ronald B. Jackson. They currently live in Sacramento, California with their son Jamal, dog YaYa, and daughter Tiffani and her five children. Jackie's son Demetrius and his family currently reside in Akron. Jackie can be reached at: jatuproductions@gmail.com

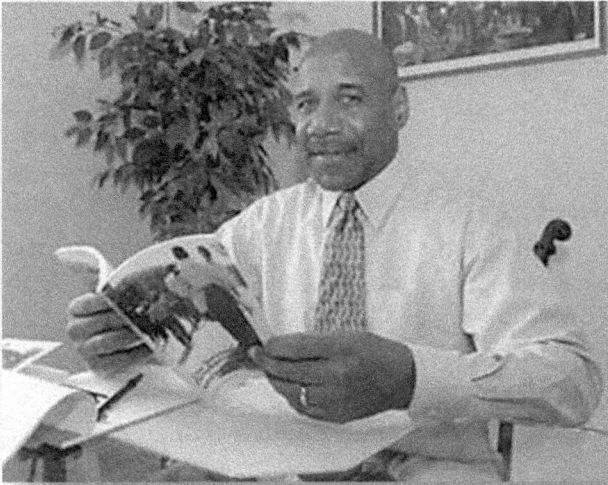

Dr. Darryl S. Tukufu

Darryl resides with his wife, Myra, outside of Memphis in Lakeland, TN. They have two sons, Ricky and Khari, and four grandchildren. An ordained Minister, he serves at Mississippi Boulevard Christian Church (Memphis). He received a B.A. degree in Social Studies from Youngstown State University, a Doctor of Ministry from Jacksonville Theological Seminary, and an M.A. in Urban Studies and a Ph.D. in Sociology from the University of Akron.

Darryl spent his first sixteen years in Cleveland, OH. He, his mother and sister then moved to Los Angeles, CA, where he soon became active in the Us Organization. He continued his involvement in a number of black cultural and activist organizations including the Committee for Unified Newark in Newark, NJ, and the

National Black Independent Political Party (NBIPP), in Akron, OH. He also worked for various affiliates of the National Urban League, and served as Executive Director of the Greater Cleveland (OH) Roundtable.

He has served in various capacities and/or faculty positions at a number of colleges and universities including in Memphis the University of Memphis, LeMoyne-Owen College, Victory University, Belhaven University, Cambridge College, Memphis Center for Urban Theological Studies (MCUTS), and Kent State (OH), Northeastern University (Boston), and Bethel University in McKenzie, TN. Darryl can be reached at jatuproductions@gmail.com